30 Days to a Healthier You: Fitness and Nutrition Plan

M U DIGINSA

ISBN: 9798877177260

ISBN: 9798877177260

DISCLAIMER

The sole intent of this eBook is to provide information. This eBook has been meticulously researched and fact-checked to the best of our ability. Nonetheless, there can be grammatical or substance errors. Also, the content in this e-book is only current as of publication. As a result, this eBook should only be used as a reference.

The objective of this eBook is to educate. The content in this e-book is not guaranteed to be accurate by the author or the publisher, and they are not liable for any mistakes or omissions.

Regarding any loss or damage caused or alleged to have been caused directly or indirectly by this eBook, the author and publisher are not liable or responsible to any person or entity.

TITLE

30 Days to a Healthier You: Fitness and Nutrition Plan

DEDICATION

To my parents, who instilled in me a love of learning and a passion for a healthier life, fitness, and nutrition plan. Your unwavering support and encouragement have driven my pursuit of knowledge and my journey to bring this book to life. Thank you for always believing in me.

And to all those who share in my passion for Healthy life, I dedicate this book to you. May it inspire, inform, and awaken a sense of wonder and excitement for all the fantastic things we have yet to discover. Let us continue to learn, grow, and explore together.

Table of Content

Introduction

Welcome to "30 Days to a Healthier You: Fitness and Nutrition Plan." Congratulations on taking the first step towards transforming your life and embarking on a 30-day journey to a healthier, more vibrant version of yourself.

It's easy to overlook the importance of prioritizing our health in the hustle and bustle of our daily lives. This book is designed to guide you through a comprehensive 30-day program focusing on two well-being pillars: fitness and nutrition. By the end of this journey, you'll feel the physical benefits but also experience a positive shift in your mindset and overall lifestyle.

Why This Program Matters:

Health is a holistic concept beyond physical fitness; it encompasses mental well-being, nutritional habits, and the harmony between mind and body. The 30-day program outlined in this book is crafted to address these aspects, providing you with a roadmap to sustainable health.

What Sets This Program Apart:

This isn't just another fitness and nutrition guide; it's a tailored plan designed to meet you where you are on your health journey. Whether you're a beginner or want to revitalize your routine, the program is flexible and adaptable.

Throughout the next 30 days, you will explore a variety of exercises, delve into the world of nutritious and delicious meals, and, most importantly, develop habits that extend beyond the program. This isn't about quick fixes or temporary changes; it's about creating a foundation for a healthier and more fulfilling life.

How to Use This Book:

- Start by assessing your current health status using the guidelines in Chapter 1.
- Create a personalized 30-day action plan with the help of Chapter 2.
- Follow the week-by-week fitness regimen outlined in Chapter 3, gradually building your strength and endurance.
- Dive into the nutritional guidelines provided in Chapter 4 and explore daily meal plans and recipes in Chapter 5.
- Confront challenges with confidence using the strategies outlined in Chapter 6.
- Track your progress, adjust, and celebrate your achievements throughout the program.
- Remember, this is your journey; the goal is progress, not perfection. Stay committed, be kind to yourself, and embrace the positive changes over the next 30 days.

Are you ready to embark on this transformative journey? Let's get started on the path to a healthier, happier you!

Chapter 1

Understanding Your Current Health Status

In the initial chapter of our transformative guide, we delve into the crucial foundation of your wellness journey: understanding your current health status. This comprehensive self-assessment will serve as the compass that guides you through the next 30 days, helping you set realistic and achievable health goals tailored to your unique needs and circumstances.

1.1 Assessing Current Fitness Levels:

Before starting any fitness program, you must clarify your current physical capabilities. This section provides simple yet effective methods to assess your fitness levels. We'll guide you through exercises and self-assessment tools, from cardiovascular endurance and strength to flexibility and balance. By understanding where you currently stand, you'll be better equipped to tailor the upcoming fitness regimen to your specific requirements, ensuring a safe and compelling journey.

Key Topics:

- Cardiovascular fitness assessment.
- Strength evaluation through basic exercises.
- Flexibility and mobility tests.
- Balance and coordination self-assessment.

1.2 Evaluating Dietary Habits:

Nutrition plays a pivotal role in achieving optimal health. In this section, we explore the intricacies of your current dietary habits. Through reflective exercises and guided questions, you'll gain insights into your eating patterns, nutritional choices, and areas needing adjustment. Understanding the role of macronutrients and micronutrients in your diet forms the basis for creating a personalized and sustainable meal plan.

Key Topics:

- Keeping a food diary for self-awareness.
- Identifying nutritional gaps and areas of improvement.
- Recognizing emotional and mindless eating habits.
- Exploring the impact of hydration on overall health.

1.3 Setting Realistic Health Goals:

Setting clear and realistic health goals is a fundamental step toward success. This section guides establishing goals that are specific, measurable, achievable, relevant, and time-bound (SMART). Whether your objectives are related to weight management, fitness milestones, or overall well-being, we'll help you articulate your aspirations and break them down into manageable steps. By the end of this chapter, you'll have a roadmap that aligns with your current health status and sets the stage for the transformative 30-day journey ahead.

Key Topics:

- Defining short-term and long-term health goals.
- Breaking down goals into actionable steps.
- Creating a timeline for goal achievement.
- Aligning goals with your values and motivations.

As you progress through Chapter 1, remember that self-awareness is the cornerstone of positive change. Embrace this opportunity to reflect, learn, and lay the groundwork for the impactful health improvements that lie ahead. Get ready to take charge of your well-being, one insightful step at a time.

Chapter 2

Creating Your 30-Day Action Plan

Welcome to the transformative journey of creating a personalized 30-day action plan that integrates fitness and nutrition seamlessly into your daily life. This chapter is your guide to design and intention, empowering you to take decisive steps toward achieving your health and wellness goals.

2.1 Designing a Personalized Fitness Routine:

Key Topics:

Identifying Preferred Workout Styles and Activities:

Understanding what types of exercise, you enjoy is crucial for long-term adherence. Discover activities that resonate with you, whether dancing, hiking, weightlifting, or yoga. This section provides insights into various workout styles and helps you find the perfect fit for your preferences.

Creating a Balanced Exercise Routine:

A well-rounded fitness routine addresses different aspects of physical health, including cardiovascular fitness, strength, flexibility, and mindfulness. Learn how to structure your weekly workouts to achieve balance and target various muscle groups for overall improvement.

Incorporating Variety to Prevent Monotony:

Variety is the spice of life, and the same holds for your fitness routine. Explore different exercises, classes, and workout formats to keep things exciting. Discover how to incorporate variety to prevent boredom and maintain motivation throughout the 30 days.

Adapting Workouts to Accommodate Your Schedule and Resources:

Life is dynamic, and so should be your fitness routine. Find out how to adjust your workouts to fit your schedule, whether you have 30 minutes or an hour. We'll also explore modifications for home workouts and those with limited equipment.

2.2 Planning a Balanced and Nutritious Diet:

Key Topics:

Understanding the Role of Carbohydrates, Proteins, and Fats:

Delve into the fundamentals of macronutrients and their role in your diet. Learn how to balance carbohydrates, proteins, and fats to support your energy levels, muscle building, and overall well-being.

Incorporating a Variety of Fruits and Vegetables:

Discover the nutritional powerhouses found in a rainbow of fruits and vegetables. We'll guide you on selecting diverse produce to ensure you receive a broad spectrum of vitamins, minerals, and antioxidants.

Exploring Lean Protein Sources and Whole Grains:

Protein is essential for muscle repair, and whole grains provide sustained energy. Explore lean protein sources and whole grains to enhance your diet's nutritional profile. Sample meal ideas will guide you in creating satisfying and nourishing meals.

Hydration Strategies for Optimal Performance:

Proper hydration is often underestimated. Understand the importance of staying hydrated and explore strategies to meet your daily fluid intake needs. Hydration plays a vital role in supporting your fitness endeavours and overall health.

2.3 Setting Achievable Milestones for the Next 30 Days:

Key Topics:

Defining Short-Term Fitness Achievements:

Establish specific fitness goals for the next 30 days, whether it's mastering a new exercise, improving endurance, or increasing flexibility, and set clear and achievable milestones to strive towards.

Establishing Dietary Milestones and Habits:

Translate your nutritional goals into actionable steps. Identify dietary habits you want to cultivate, such as mindful eating, meal prepping, or reducing sugar intake. Learn how to establish practices that contribute to your long-term well-being.

Tracking Progress Through Journals and Apps:

Discover practical ways to track your fitness and nutrition progress. Whether through journaling, apps, or wearable devices, monitoring your achievements and challenges provides valuable insights. Learn how tracking enhances self-awareness and motivates continued effort.

Celebrating Victories Along the Way:

Every small success deserves celebration. Acknowledge and celebrate your achievements, no matter how minor. Positive reinforcement is crucial in maintaining motivation and fostering a positive mindset throughout your 30-day journey.

As you immerse yourself in the detailed exploration of these critical topics, envision the 30 days ahead as a canvas for positive change. Your action plan is not just a list of tasks; it's a dynamic blueprint crafted to guide you toward a healthier and more vibrant version of yourself. The journey begins now.

Chapter 3

Week-by-Week Fitness Regimen

Embark on a four-week journey of transformative fitness as we delve into a structured week-by-week regimen. Each week is meticulously crafted to target different aspects of your physical well-being, ensuring a holistic and progressive approach to your health. Let's dive into the specific focus and critical topics for each week.

Week 1: Introduction to Exercise - Building a Foundation

Key Topics:

Sample Workouts for Beginners:

This week is all about laying the groundwork for your fitness journey. Explore beginner-friendly workouts designed to introduce you to various movements and exercise formats. From bodyweight exercises to simple strength-building routines, these workouts are tailored to your starting point.

Importance of Warm-Up and Cool-Down Exercises:

Understanding the significance of warming up and cooling down is crucial for injury prevention and overall performance. Learn dynamic warm-up exercises to prepare your body for activity and effective cool-down stretches to aid muscle recovery and flexibility.

Week 2: Cardiovascular Conditioning

Key Topics:

Exploring Cardio Exercises for Endurance:

Cardiovascular health is the focus of Week 2. Discover a variety of cardio exercises that elevate your heart rate, improve endurance, and boost overall cardiovascular fitness. From brisk walks to high-intensity interval training (HIIT), explore options that align with your fitness level.

Incorporating Variety into Workouts:

Avoid monotony by introducing variety into your cardio routines. We'll discuss different types of cardio exercises and how to incorporate them into your weekly regimen. Variety not only keeps things exciting but also challenges other muscle groups.

Week 3: Strength Training for a Toned Body

Key Topics:

Introduction to Strength Training:

Week 3 marks the introduction to strength training, a crucial component for overall fitness. Understand the principles of strength training, its benefits, and why it's essential to a well-rounded fitness routine.

Bodyweight Exercises and Basic Weightlifting:

Explore the world of bodyweight exercises that build functional strength. Additionally, we'll introduce basic weightlifting techniques focusing on proper form and safety. Whether you're using dumbbells or barbells, this week is about sculpting and toning your body.

Week 4: Flexibility and Mind-Body Connection

Key Topics:

Incorporating Yoga and Stretching:

Flexibility and the mind-body connection take center stage in Week 4. Learn the fundamentals of yoga and explore stretching exercises that enhance flexibility and promote relaxation. These practices improve posture and reduce muscle tension and overall well-being.

Stress Management Techniques:

Understand the profound impact of stress on your health and discover techniques to manage and alleviate stress. Mindfulness, breathing exercises, and other stress-relief practices will be integrated into your fitness routine, fostering a holistic connection between your body and mind.

Remember that consistency and gradual progression are essential as you progress each week. Listen to your body, celebrate small victories, and embrace each week's evolving strength and vitality. Your four-week fitness regimen is a stepping stone toward a healthier and more resilient you. Let's commence this empowering journey together!

Chapter 4

Nutritional Guidelines for a Healthy Lifestyle

Welcome to a pivotal chapter dedicated to unravelling nutrition mysteries and empowering you to make informed and nourishing choices for your well-being. In "Nutritional Guidelines for a Healthy Lifestyle," we'll explore the fundamental building blocks of nutrition, guide you in creating a balanced meal plan, and provide delicious and wholesome snack options to support your health journey.

Key Topics:

4.1 Understanding Macronutrients and Micronutrients:

- Macronutrients: The Foundations of Nutrition
- Carbohydrates: Unveil the role of carbohydrates and their diverse sources in providing energy, from whole grains to fruits.
- Proteins: Explore the importance of proteins for muscle repair and growth and discover lean sources for a balanced diet.
- Fats: Delve into the world of healthy fats, understanding their role in hormone production and overall well-being.
- Micronutrients: The Power of the Minuscule

- Vitamins and Minerals: Navigate the rich landscape of essential vitamins and minerals, discovering their functions and food sources.
- Antioxidants: Uncover the protective properties of antioxidants and how they contribute to cellular health.

4.2 Designing a Balanced Meal Plan:

Building Blocks of a Nourishing Meal:

- Balancing Macronutrients: Learn to create meals that harmoniously combine carbohydrates, proteins, and fats to meet your nutritional needs.
- Portion Control: Understand the importance of portion sizes to avoid overeating and support weight management goals.
- Sample Meal Plans (Breakfast, Lunch, and Dinner Ideas): Explore sample meal plans that cater to diverse tastes and dietary preferences, from plant-based to omnivorous options.

4.3 Healthy Snack Options:

Snacking with Purpose:

- Nutrient-Dense Snacking: Discover snacks that provide a nutritional boost while satisfying cravings, promoting sustained energy throughout the day.
- Mindful Snacking: Understand the importance of mindful eating, emphasizing the connection between your body's hunger cues and food choices.

Snack Ideas for Every Occasion:

- Pre-Workout Snacks: Fuel your workouts with pre-exercise snack ideas that enhance energy and performance.
- Post-Workout Recovery: Explore post-workout snacks that support muscle recovery and replenish glycogen stores.
- As you navigate the nutritional landscape in this chapter, remember that your relationship with food is a vital aspect of overall health. By understanding the roles of macronutrients and micronutrients, designing balanced meals, and making mindful snack choices, you're laying the groundwork for sustained well-being. Let the journey to a healthier lifestyle unfold through informed and empowered nutritional decisions.

Chapter 5

Daily Meal Plans and Recipes

Welcome to the heart of your nutrition journey! In this chapter, we will take the principles discussed in the previous chapter and translate them into actionable and delicious daily meal plans. Get ready to explore various simple, nutritious recipes designed to fuel your body throughout the 30-day program. Let's embark on a culinary adventure that supports your health goals and tantalizes your taste buds.

Key Topics:

5.1 Providing Daily Meal Plans for the 30 days:

Understanding the Structure of Daily Meal Plans:

- Balancing Nutrients: Each meal plan is meticulously crafted to ensure a balanced intake of macronutrients (carbohydrates, proteins, and fats) and micronutrients (vitamins and minerals).
- Adaptability: Meal plans are adaptable to various dietary preferences, including vegetarian, vegan, and omnivorous options.
- Portion Considerations: Portion sizes are carefully considered to meet your energy needs without overindulgence.

5.2 Simple and Nutritious Recipes for Breakfast:

Breakfast: The Energizing Start:

- Protein-Packed Breakfasts: Explore recipes that kickstart your day with protein-rich options, promoting satiety and sustained energy.
- Fiber-Focused Choices: Incorporate high-fibre ingredients to support digestive health and keep you feeling full.

5.3 Simple and Nutritious Recipes for Lunch:

Lunch: The Midday Sustenance:

- Wholesome Salad Creations: Dive into vibrant salads with various flavors and nutrients.
- Protein-Packed Lunches: Discover satisfying lunch options featuring lean proteins and various colourful vegetables.

5.4 Simple and Nutritious Recipes for Dinner:

Dinner: The Nourishing Finale:

- Balanced Dinner Plates: Explore well-rounded recipes that balance proteins, whole grains, and vegetables.
- Quick and Nutrient-Dense Dinners: Incorporate easy-to-prepare recipes for busy evenings without compromising nutrition.

5.5 Simple and Nutritious Recipes for Snacks:

Snacks: Nourishing Moments Between Meals:

- Healthy Snack Options: Enjoy a selection of snacks that curb cravings while providing essential nutrients.
- Snack Preparation Tips: Learn how to prepare snacks in advance for convenient and mindful consumption.

5.6 Culinary Variety for the 30-Day Journey:

Exploring Culinary Diversity:

- Cultural Cuisine Inspirations: Infuse variety into your meals by exploring recipes inspired by different cultures.
- Ingredient Substitutions: Learn how to make ingredient substitutions to accommodate dietary preferences and restrictions.

As you journey through the daily meal plans and recipes in this chapter, remember that nourishing your body is not just about sustenance; it's an opportunity to savor flavors, embrace variety, and foster a positive relationship with food. Let the joy of wholesome and delicious meals accompany you throughout the 30-day program, making every bite a celebration of your commitment to a healthier lifestyle.

Chapter 6

Overcoming Challenges

Congratulations on reaching Chapter 6! As you embark on your 30-day journey, it's crucial to acknowledge that challenges are a natural part of any transformative process. This chapter tackles common obstacles head-on, providing strategies to navigate setbacks, stay motivated, and cultivate a positive mindset. Let's build resilience together and ensure that nothing stands in your path to a healthier you.

Key Topics:

6.1 Addressing Common Obstacles During the 30-Day Journey:

Anticipating and Overcoming Challenges:

- Time Constraints: Explore time-efficient strategies for fitting workouts and nutritious meals into a busy schedule.
- Social and Peer Influences: Navigate social situations and peer dynamics that may challenge your health goals.
- Travel and Dining Out: Learn how to make mindful choices when traveling or dining out, ensuring you stay on track with your 30-day program.

6.2 Motivational Strategies for Consistency:

Cultivating Sustainable Motivation:

- Setting Personal Milestones: Establish short-term and long-term milestones to keep your motivation high throughout the journey.
- Accountability Partnerships: Explore the benefits of having a workout buddy or a nutrition accountability partner to share the journey with.

Staying Inspired:

- Inspirational Stories: Draw inspiration from the success stories of others who have overcome challenges on their wellness journeys.
- Visualization Techniques: Utilize visualization exercises to envision your success and reinforce your commitment to the 30-day program.

6.3 Encouraging a Positive Mindset:

Fostering a Positive Perspective:

- Embracing Progress Over Perfection: Shift your focus from perfection to progress, celebrating each step forward, no matter how small.
- Practicing Gratitude: Cultivate gratitude for the positive changes in your life, enhancing your overall well-being.
- Self-Compassion: Develop a compassionate mindset towards yourself, acknowledging that setbacks are growth opportunities.

Coping with Setbacks:

- Learning from Challenges: Understand that setbacks are part of the journey and opportunities to learn and readjust.
- Adapting and Moving Forward: Develop resilience by adapting to challenges and maintaining momentum in the face of setbacks.

As you navigate the challenges presented in this chapter, remember that transformation is a journey, not a destination. By proactively addressing obstacles, staying motivated, and fostering a positive mindset, you're building a foundation for sustainable health and well-being. Embrace the process, celebrate your victories, and keep moving forward with confidence and resilience. You've got this!

Chapter 7

Assessing Progress and Adjustments

Welcome to a pivotal chapter where we shift our focus from the beginning of the journey to a reflection on the strides you've made. In "Assessing Progress and Adjustments," we explore the art of self-reflection, tracking your achievements, and making informed adjustments to ensure your wellness journey remains tailored to your evolving needs. Get ready to celebrate successes, acknowledge growth, and fine-tune your path to a healthier, more vibrant you.

Key Topics:

7.1 Tracking Fitness Improvements:

Celebrating Milestones:

- Strength and Endurance Gains: Recognize improvements in your strength and endurance through benchmarks such as increased weights, longer workout durations, or enhanced performance in specific exercises.
- Flexibility and Mobility: Acknowledge gains in flexibility and mobility, appreciating the increased range of motion and reduced stiffness.

Measuring Cardiovascular Fitness:

- Progress in Cardiovascular Endurance: Track improvements in cardiovascular fitness by noting increased stamina during cardio exercises, quicker recovery times, and improved heart rate variability.

7.2 Monitoring Changes in Energy Levels and Mood:

Energy Levels as an Indicator:

- Observing Day-to-Day Energy Levels: Notice changes in your daily energy levels, understanding how they relate to your fitness routine, sleep quality, and nutrition.
- Morning and Evening Comparisons: Assess variations in energy levels between mornings and evenings, identifying patterns and adjusting your daily schedule accordingly.

Mood as a Reflection of Well-Being:

- Noting Positive Mood Changes: Recognize the impact of regular exercise and a balanced diet on your mood, stress levels, and overall emotional well-being.
- Identifying Stressors and Coping Strategies: Evaluate stressors in your life and recognize effective coping mechanisms, ensuring a holistic approach to well-being.

7.3 Adjusting the Plan Based on Individual Needs:

Personalizing Your 30-Day Journey:

- Reflecting on Preferences: Assess your preferences and enjoyment levels in various exercises and meals, making adjustments to keep the journey engaging.
- Adapting to Lifestyle Changes: Modify your plan to accommodate changes in your schedule, responsibilities, or personal circumstances.

Fine-Tuning Nutrition:

- Exploring Nutritional Adjustments: Evaluate the impact of your meal plan on energy levels, satiety, and overall satisfaction. Adjust align with your nutritional preferences and requirements.

Unlocking Your Potential:

In this chapter, we unleash the power of self-reflection and adjustment—a dynamic process that propels you forward on your health journey. Imagine celebrating newfound strength, revealing in an improved mood, and customizing your plan to suit your needs. This is the chapter where you become the architect of your wellness destiny.

The Symphony of Progress:

Your body is a symphony, and every workout, every nutrient, every positive shift contributes to the masterpiece of your well-being. Explore the nuances of your symphony, and let this chapter be the crescendo that elevates your journey.

Your Journey, Your Rules:

It's time to break free from one-size-fits-all approaches. This chapter empowers you to sculpt your 30-day plan into a masterpiece that resonates with your rhythm, preferences, and aspirations. Brace yourself for a branch that turns progress assessment into art and adjustments into a personalized masterpiece. Your journey, your rules—let the exploration begin!

Chapter 8

Life Beyond the 30 Days

Congratulations on reaching the culmination of your 30-day journey! As you stand at the threshold of this chapter, it's not just an end but a new beginning—a gateway to a life where health, vitality, and well-being become enduring companions. In "Life Beyond the 30 Days," we'll guide you through the transition into a sustainable, long-term, healthy lifestyle, help you set new fitness and nutrition goals, and inspire you to continue this transformative journey with unwavering commitment.

Key Topics:

8.1 Transitioning into a Sustainable, Long-Term Healthy Lifestyle:

Embedding Habits for Life:

- Building Sustainable Routines: Learn how to transform the positive habits cultivated in the past 30 days into lasting lifestyle changes.

- Mindful Decision-Making: Embrace mindfulness in your daily choices, from meal planning to physical activities, ensuring sustained health benefits.

Cultivating Consistency:

- Consistency Over Perfection: Shift your focus from short-term perfection to long-term consistency, understanding that sustainable health is a journey, not a destination.

- Adapting to Lifestyle Changes: Explore strategies to integrate health-conscious choices into evolving life circumstances seamlessly.

8.2 Setting New Fitness and Nutrition Goals:

Elevating Your Aspirations:

- Reflecting on Achievements: Celebrate the milestones achieved during the 30-day program, allowing them to inspire and fuel your future goals.

- Defining New Fitness Milestones: Articulate fresh fitness objectives that align with your evolving aspirations and capabilities.

Nurturing Nutrition Objectives:

- Exploring Culinary Exploration: Continue the culinary journey by experimenting with new recipes and ingredients that align with your nutritional goals.

- Fine-Tuning Dietary Preferences: Adjust your meal plan based on personal preferences, exploring new ways to nourish your body while savouring various flavours.

8.3 Encouraging Readers to Continue Their Journey:

Embracing the Ongoing Transformation:

- Inspiration for the Long Haul: Draw inspiration from the transformations witnessed in the past 30 days, realizing that this is just the beginning of a lifelong wellness journey.

- Connecting with a Supportive Community: Seek and foster connections within communities with similar health goals, finding encouragement and motivation in shared experiences.

Empowering the Mindset:

- Embracing a Growth Mindset: Cultivate a growth mindset that perceives challenges as opportunities for learning and growth, fostering resilience in the face of obstacles.

- Acknowledging the Journey's Fluid Nature: Understand that the health journey is dynamic, with continuous learning and adaptation being integral components.

Beyond the Finish Line:

This chapter is not a conclusion; it's a launchpad into a future where health is not a destination but a perpetual exploration. As you stand at the crossroads, envision the endless possibilities of your ongoing journey—a life where each day is an opportunity to enhance your well-being.

Setting Sail for New Horizons:

Unfurl the sails of newfound strength, resilience, and knowledge as you navigate the seas of lifelong health. Let this chapter be the compass that guides you toward new horizons filled with vitality, purpose and the promise of continued transformation.

Your Journey, Your Legacy:

Your 30-day journey is a chapter in the epic novel of your life. As you turn the page to "Life Beyond the 30 Days," remember that the narrative is still unfolding, and the pen is in your hands. The choices you make today will influence the chapters yet to be written. Your journey, your legacy—may it be a tale of resilience, growth, and the unwavering pursuit of a healthier, more fulfilling life. Onward!

Conclusion:

As we draw the final curtain on this transformative 30-day journey, take a moment to reflect on the incredible odyssey you've undertaken. From the first steps to the challenges overcome, you've navigated through a comprehensive program designed to elevate your well-being. In this conclusion, let's revisit the essence of the past 30 days, celebrate your remarkable achievements, and reinforce the importance of maintaining a steadfast commitment to your health.

Recap of the 30-Day Program:

The past 30 days have been a symphony of self-discovery, discipline, and growth. You've engaged in purposeful workouts, embraced nourishing meals, and delved into the intricacies of a healthier lifestyle. From understanding the fundamentals of fitness and nutrition to crafting personalized meal plans, each day was a step toward a stronger, more vibrant version of yourself.

Through chapters that explored various facets of well-being—physical, mental, and emotional—you've gathered tools to sculpt a lifestyle that fosters resilience, mindfulness, and lasting vitality. The program wasn't just about the exercises or the meals; it was about redefining your relationship with health and laying the foundation for a sustainable, lifelong commitment to well-being.

Celebrating Achievements and Progress:

Now, let's revel in the triumphs you've achieved. Celebrate the moments when you pushed your physical limits, the times you chose nourishing foods that fueled your body, and the instances when you embraced challenges as opportunities for growth. Whether it's the increased weights, the enhanced flexibility, or the newfound joy in mindful eating, every achievement contributes to the masterpiece of your well-being, no matter how small.

Take pride in the commitment you've shown to your health, the consistency you've cultivated, and the resilience that carried you through the highs and lows of the journey. You are not just closing a chapter; you are etching a legacy—a testament to your dedication to a healthier, happier life.

Encouraging Readers to Maintain a Commitment to Their Health:

As this chapter concludes, it's essential to recognize that your health journey is an ongoing narrative. The 30 days were a launchpad, a catalyst for change, but the story doesn't end here. The habits you've formed, the lessons you've learned, and the transformations you've witnessed are the seeds of a flourishing future.

Maintaining a commitment to your health is not about perfection but the consistent pursuit of well-being. Continue to set realistic goals, adapt your routines to suit your evolving lifestyle, and nurture a positive mindset. Embrace the fluid nature of your journey, knowing that each day is an opportunity to reaffirm your commitment to a healthier, more fulfilling life.

Remember, you are the author of your health story. Every choice you make, every step you take, contributes to the narrative. As you move forward, carry the strength, knowledge, and resilience cultivated during these 30 days. Your journey is a testament to your capacity for growth, and the path ahead is illuminated by the radiance of your commitment to a life filled with vitality and well-being.

Thank you for embarking on this journey with dedication and enthusiasm. Here's to your health, your growth, and the limitless possibilities that lie ahead. Onward to the next chapter!

Appendix:

Congratulations on completing the transformative journey outlined in this guide! As you continue your pursuit of health and well-being, this appendix is a valuable resource hub. Explore additional materials, find answers to frequently asked questions, and connect with further resources to support your ongoing journey.

FAQs Related to Fitness and Nutrition:

Q1: Can I customize the fitness routine based on my fitness level?

A1: Absolutely! The provided fitness routine serves as a foundation. Feel free to modify exercises, weights, or intensity based on your capabilities.

Q2: How can I handle cravings for unhealthy snacks?

A2: Try incorporating healthier alternatives, such as fruit or nuts, into your meal plan. Also, stay hydrated, as thirst can sometimes be mistaken for hunger.

Q3: What if I miss a workout or indulge in an unhealthy meal?

A3: Remember, consistency is key, but occasional deviations are expected. Acknowledge, learn from, and continue your routine without guilt.

Thank you!

Thank you for choosing this guide as your companion to a healthier you. We're here to support you in every step of your journey. Wishing you continued success, growth, and well-being!